Vegan Lean

Get a Slim Body, All Day Energy, and Glow with Happiness with a Vegan Lifestyle

Inspiring Real Success Stories and a
5 Day Meal Plan Guide for Faster Weight Loss Results

Caleesi Giovo

© 2016 by Caleesi Giovo - All rights reserved.

This document is geared towards providing exact and reliable information in regards to the topic and issue covered. The publication is sold with the idea that the publisher is not required to render accounting, officially permitted, or otherwise, qualified services. If advice is necessary, legal or professional, a practiced individual in the profession should be ordered.

- From a Declaration of Principles which was accepted and approved equally by a Committee of the American Bar Association and a Committee of Publishers and Associations.

In no way is it legal to reproduce, duplicate, or transmit any part of this document in either electronic means or in printed format. Recording of this publication is strictly prohibited and any storage of this document is not allowed unless with written permission from the publisher. All rights reserved.

The information provided herein is stated to be truthful and consistent, in that any liability, in terms of inattention or otherwise, by any usage or abuse of any policies, processes, or directions contained within is the solitary and utter responsibility of the recipient reader. Under no circumstances will any legal responsibility or blame be held against the publisher for any reparation, damages, or monetary loss due to the information herein, either directly or indirectly.

Respective authors own all copyrights not held by the publisher.

The information herein is offered for informational purposes solely, and is universal as so. The presentation of the information is without contract or any type of guarantee assurance.

The trademarks that are used are without any consent, and the publication of the trademark is without permission or backing by the trademark owner. All trademarks and brands within this book are for clarifying purposes only and are the owned by the owners themselves, not affiliated with this document.

CONTENTS

01: BEING VEGAN LEAN AND HOW TO CREATE IT

Benefits of a Vegan Lifestyle and It's Growing Popularity. 1
How Eating Vegan is Easy for Long Term Weight Loss 4
Foods that Turn Your Body into a Super Fat Burner
and Metabolism Booster 13

02: AVOID COMMON MISTAKES AND GET THE BEST RESULTS

Eating Vegan to Get Happy, Focused, and Productive 17
Eating Vegan: Do's and Don'ts 21
5 Tips for Weight Loss to Get Vegan Lean 31

03: PUTTING IT INTO ACTION

5 Day Meal Plan Guide for Faster Results 33
    Day 1 35
    Day 2 37
    Day 3 39
    Day 4 41
    Day 5 43

BONUS: How to Stop Food Cravings in Less than
    5 Minutes! 45

INTRODUCTION

I want to thank you and congratulate you for buying the book, Vegan Lean.

This book contains proven steps and strategies on how to adopt a vegan diet to promote weight loss and a healthy lifestyle.

Vegan Lean is an insightful guide to vegan weight loss that will guide you through building a healthy meal plan and avoiding common mistakes to maximize the benefits of a high carb, low fat plant-based diet focused on whole, nutritious foods.

Thanks again for buying this book. I hope you enjoy it!

BENEFITS OF A VEGAN LIFESTYLE AND IT'S GROWING POPULARITY

Once upon a time, saying "I'm vegan" was a statement that would cause a bit of concerned eyebrow raising from friends and family members. To the general public, it likely brought up images of red-paint-throwing extremists or a long-haired couple named Rain and Lotus Flower living under an organic apple tree with their goat named Jude.

Today it's a different story.

With the growing endorsement of a plant-based diet from athletes, celebrities, and nutrition experts, veganism is finally gaining the mainstream attention it deserves as an ideal dietary choice for those looking to lose weight for the long haul and enjoy a happier, healthier life.

However, going vegan is certainly not just the latest fad diet. It is so much more than that. Veganism is an easy lifestyle choice that is great for our bodies, the environment, and our many animal friends.

This book will offer step-by-step guidance for an easy transition into a vegan diet that will help you:

- Know the right vegan foods for permanent weight loss
- Choose foods that boost your metabolism
- Get all day energy (no more afternoon crashes!)
- Improve your skin, hair, and mental focus (and overall health)
- Maintain a slim body
- Avoid common mistakes

Success Stories: 240lbs Gone on a Vegan Diet

Jerry Monesmith

After trying the South Beach Diet, Atkins, and many other weight loss programs with little results, Jerry knew he had to transition his lifestyle after seeing one of his friends having success weight loss with a vegan lifestyle. Sticking with a vegan lifestyle with mostly high carb, low fat, whole foods allowed him to loose over 200 lbs. and shocked his family and friends. He loves this lifestyle so much that he'll never go back. Check out his weight loss story and what he eats on his YouTube interview:

http://bit.ly/24DSfUc

HOW EATING VEGAN IS EASY FOR LONG TERM WEIGHT LOSS

A vegan diet doesn't mean you are sentenced to eating only carrots and lettuce for the rest of your days. In fact, the growing popularity of a plant-based diet means that restaurants, supermarkets, and even food trucks are providing more vegan options than ever.

When starting out as a vegan, however, it is important to understand that there are certain dietary guidelines to consider that will help you to maximize your health and promote weight loss.

The best way to boost the benefits of a vegan diet is to eat a whole food based, high carb diet while avoiding refined sugar, excess fat, high amounts sodium, and processed food.

Loading Up on Fruits and Veggies to Stay Slim

It turns out Mom was right to make you eat your vegetables. Both vegans and meat eaters should be eating plenty of fruits and veggies, but cutting animal products gives your diet extra room to eat more of them.

The best part is that you can eat as much as you want and still easily reach your goal weight. Your body loves the natural nutrients in fruits and vegetables. When your body gets the nutrients it needs, it has the energy to become a super fat burner.

Here's a hint: for faster weight loss, aim to have 70% or more plant-based foods in your daily diet. This works best when you also limit oils, nuts, seeds, avocados, and other fats to 20% or less of your calories each day (even if they are considered "healthy fats").

How Eating (Whole Grain) Bread Speeds Up Your Metabolism

Whole grains packed with healthy carbs and fiber keep you energized and full while on a vegan diet. What your Atkins and Paleo addicted friends don't know is that a high carbohydrate diet actually speeds your metabolism and makes it easier to lose weight.

When your body doesn't have enough carbs, it starts to burn muscle tissue, which is what keeps your metabolism fast and body looking lean. The more muscle you have, the faster your metabolism will be (and the better your clothing will fit).

The best way to know how "whole" your grains are is to look for products with a short ingredient list, little or no additives, and a high fiber content. An added bonus is that whole grains can also be a good source of protein!

To get the most out of a high carb vegan diet, and keep that metabolism going strong, choose whole grains such as:

- Brown rice
- Sprouted grains
- Whole wheat
- Quinoa
- Couscous
- Oats

Unlike white bread and processed grains that are filled with empty calories, these whole grains are high in fiber and energizing carbohydrates, both of which will keep you full for longer and promote weight loss.

How do Vegans Get their Protein?

This is one of the most common questions asked by meat-eating skeptics. To a person who has been raised to believe that meat is the only kind of protein out there, veganism might look like a difficult or even dangerous dietary choice. However, nothing could be further from the truth.

Many people actually eat too much protein, which can be even more damaging to your body. Eating a diet that is over 35% protein, especially when you don't eat enough carbs, can lead to the buildup of acids called ketones. Ketones are toxic substances made when your body starts to use its own fat cells for energy after it runs out of carbs.

The idea of your body burning fat for energy might sound good, but it's not that simple. Ketones can really harm the kidneys as they try to remove these toxins and can cause chemical imbalances in your blood. [1]

---

[1] http://www.medicinenet.com/how_much_dietary_protein_to_consume-page2/views.htm

Instead of eating way too much animal protein, vegans eat a healthy amount of protein from wholesome plant sources. Some of the best vegan proteins include:

- Lentils
- Beans
- Soy
- Tempeh
- Seitan
- Leafy greens
- Seeds and small amounts of nuts

Lose the Fat to Lose Your Fat

When eating a vegan diet, it is important to watch your fat and sodium intake, as overdoing it on either one, will slow down weight loss progress. Eating some healthy fats is incredibly important for the absorption of nutrients, but it shouldn't make up more than 20% of your diet, especially if you are looking to lose some body fat.

While nuts, avocados, and peanut butter are nutrient-dense whole foods, they are packed with calories and should be enjoyed in small portions as a part of a meal rather than a stand-alone snack.

Excess fat (particularly animal fats) in the diet causes buildup in the body's cells, which creates insulin blockages. Insulin allows sugar to come into your cells and energize your muscles. A low-fat diet keeps insulin issues at bay, which keeps your cells healthy.[2]

Sodium can also slow weight loss as too much of it will cause your body to retain water, making you feel puffy and bloated. Avoiding processed foods will help to cut both fat and salt significantly.

Try not to be heavy-handed when adding oils and salts while cooking at home. Instead, add lots of spices, herbs, and fresh ingredients to ensure that your meals are bursting with flavor.

B12 is Brain Food

One important nutrient that humans need is B12, which is essential for proper nervous system and brain function. Most people get B12 by eating animal products, so vegans should take special care to make sure they add it to their diet.

---

[2] http://www.aspeninstitute.org/about/blog/dr-neal-barnard-pitches-physical-mental-benefits-vegan-diet

The most common ways that vegans do this is by taking a daily B12 supplement or adding nutritional yeast to their foods, which is an ingredient often sprinkled on pasta, vegetables, or tofu for a delicious, buttery flavor.

Avoid a Snack Attack

Be aware that the popularity of a vegan diet has resulted in a greater variety of unhealthy vegan snack foods. Even though meat-free corn dogs and Oreos are vegan doesn't mean you should be eating them every day.

One of the best ways to avoid overeating on snacks is to make sure you're filling up on plenty of plant-based foods. Make sure that you have plenty of fruits and vegetables in your fridge and freezer so you can easily reach for them when hunger strikes.

If you're looking to lose weight, it's important to remember that vegan snack food is still snack food, and even though animal products have been eliminated, they likely have plenty of sugar, fat, and sodium to sabotage your health goals.

Be Kind to Yourself

That being said, a vegan diet should help you to be more compassionate not only to animals but to yourself as well. Balance and moderation are the most important factors of a sustainable, healthy lifestyle.

While it's important to focus on healthy eating, we're not nutrition robots. We are normal people.

No one can be 100% perfect all of the time, and it's up to you to listen to the signals that your body is sending and to honor them. You might be surprised to find that your body actually loves eating all of that quinoa and kale.

Success Stories: The Banana Girl

Freelee

Struggling with her weight for years, Freelee came from a background of anorexia, bulimia, binge eating, drugs, and weight loss stimulants. Her body fought back and she gained over 40 lbs. She now is a raving fan of a high carb, low-fat vegan lifestyle and loves her energy levels, happy mood, and slim body while eating 30 bananas a day sometimes. Check out her tips on a vegan lifestyle for permanent weight loss:

http://bit.ly/1SYOeif

FOODS THAT TURN YOUR BODY INTO A SUPER FAT BURNER AND METABOLISM BOOSTER

The adoption a plant-based lifestyle will do so much more for your body than just aiding in weight loss. Vegans who enjoy a diet consisting of high carb, whole foods experience lots of added health benefits simply by eliminating animal products, including:

- Improved digestion for faster fat burning
- More energy for a booming metabolism
- Higher levels of vitamins that keep the body healthy and slim

Let Food Move You

Animal products are difficult for the body to convert into energy and take a serious toll on your digestion (anyone who has eaten too many grilled cheese sandwiches can relate). Plant-based foods are often high in fiber, which is great for your digestive organs and helps to fight colon cancer.

Super Foods for Super Health

Eating a diet of only whole, plant-based foods also increases the number of vitamins that you eat, which means better overall health for your body.

A balanced vegan diet includes amazing mood-boosting nutrients like magnesium, potassium, folate, antioxidants, vitamin C, vitamin E, and phytochemicals, all of which are going to make your body feel much better than pizza and burgers ever would.

Not only will all that nutrient-filled goodness help you feel good now, but will help you in the long run, especially with maintaining a slim body.

A vegan diet can lower your risk of heart disease, arthritis, osteoporosis, high blood pressure and cholesterol, diabetes, certain cancers, and cardiovascular disease.[3]

Eat More and Weigh Less

Do you feel completely zapped of energy after eating a cheeseburger or pizza? There's actually a reason for that.

Consuming fatty, artery clogging, and often toxic animal products weigh you down and keep your body from running efficiently.

A diet high in complex vegan carbs provides your body with nutrient-dense fuel to keep you energized without causing long term damage to your system.[4] Also, those who eliminate animal products have a faster metabolism.

Vegans burn calories up to sixteen percent faster than meat eaters for a minimum of three hours after eating, meaning you can eat more food and weigh less!

---

[3] http://www.nursingdegree.net/blog/19/57-health-benefits-of-going-vegan/

[4] http://www.vegetariantimes.com/article/why-go-veg-learn-about-becoming-a-vegetarian/

While fitting into your skinny jeans is certainly an enticing reason to commit to a plant-based lifestyle, eating vegan is also a wise investment in your long term health. All of the amazing physical benefits of a wholesome vegan diet will allow you to live your life to the fullest with tons of energy and a happy, healthy body.

Success Stories: 30lb. Weight Loss on Unlimited Calories

Nutrition by Victoria

Experimenting with various dieting approaches (low carb/high protein diets, vegetarian, vegan, raw, fasting) in an attempt to improve her weight, she finally found the high carb, low-fat vegan lifestyle. At first she gained weight because of metabolic damage from constant undereating. 3 years later she still enjoys the amazing benefits of 2500 to 4000 calories a day and 30 lbs. slimmer! Check out her weight loss transformation pictures:

http://bit.ly/1T5EDZo

EATING VEGAN TO GET HAPPY, FOCUSED, AND PRODUCTIVE

There's a reason your vegan friend is always cheerful, and it's not because she's the "glass half full" type. A plant-based diet has been proven to positively affect your brain chemistry, and studies show that eating more fruits and vegetables reduces anxiety and boosts your mood. Vitamins found in plant sources like calcium, iron, chromium, folate, magnesium are all proven to improve mood and reduce stress.[5]

Meat is a Mood Killer

While eating steak might make you feel good temporarily, you're setting yourself up for some major crankiness later.

---

[5] http://greatist.com/happiness/nutrients-boost-mood

In a study published in Nutrition Journal, the consumption of animal fats by participants resulted in mood disturbances, while eating vegan showed increased feelings of happiness.[6]

Plus, committing to a diet that promotes animal rights and environmental sustainability gives you even more reasons to feel good at the end of the day.

Eat Vegan and Get Smart

Eating vegan not only makes you happy but more focused and productive as well. The vitamins in whole, vegan foods help you to think more clearly.

Just like the body's other critical organs, our brains need plenty of nourishment for proper functioning. Foods that aid mental focus include leafy greens, berries, and whole grains.

Additionally, our brain cells crave and need natural sugars found in fruits and vegetables. Natural sugar is the brain's preferred source of energy. Consuming natural sugar

---

[6] http://healthyeating.sfgate.com/being-vegetarian-affect-mood-3193.html

improves memory, focus, and cognitive thinking.[7] So when you think you're dying for a cupcake, your brain is probably asking for an apple instead!

While giving up addictive, over-processed foods may seem hard at first, you will quickly notice that you actually enjoy eating foods that keep you satisfied and nourished. In fact, the more frequently you eat nutrient-dense foods, the more you will begin to crave them as your body begins to recognize how amazing they make you feel.

After eating vegan, you'll begin to notice how unappetizing meat, dairy, and other animal products begin to look. And junk food will start to look like, well... junk. More likely than not, an omnivorous lifestyle will be a distant, less-than-fond memory that you will not ever choose to revisit.

---

[7] http://www.webmd.com/add-adhd/ss/slideshow-brain-foods-that-help-you-concentrate

Success Stories: "Finally Hit My Goal Weight!"

Christine Magnarelli

For the longest time, Christine struggled with binge eating late at night on her favorite junk foods like cookies, Twix bars, and any other fatty sweets she could find at the convenience store. After being inspired by Freelee, as well as some other nutritionist, she started to eat mostly fruits and vegetables. After struggling for years to lose the extra ten pounds, it easily fell off while eating more calories! Plus maintaining her desired weight has been easy to maintain.

powerovercravings.com

EATING VEGAN: DO'S AND DON'TS

Committing to a vegan diet is certainly a transition that requires a little wisdom and guidance for beginners. Without proper planning and sensible precautions, some people may give up too quickly or claim veganism has undesirable effects.

By honoring the following guidelines, you can avoid common pitfalls and easily adopt a vegan diet that will help you feel lighter, happier, and healthier.

Vegan Do's

Build a Foundation from Whole Foods

- **Do eat mostly fruits and vegetables.**
  They are packed with nutrients and will keep you satisfied on a vegan diet.

- **Do eat plenty of carbs for high energy and metabolism power.**
  A diet too low in carbs will zap your energy and leave you in a constant state of hunger. Whole grains and fruits are your best sources for carbohydrates.

- **Do have many whole foods as possible in your house at all times.**
  Purchase local and organic products whenever possible. Plus, having healthy food always in stock helps when cravings come on.

- **Do stay hydrated all day.**
  This keeps your body functioning properly and helps you to digest foods high in fiber. Aim for two liters of water per day.

Keep your diet balanced

- **Do balance your meals with natural plant protein.**
  This keeps your muscles strong.

- **Do keep your fat intake under 20% of your daily calories.**
  It's important to eat enough fat, but too much of it will add excess calories to your diet and keep you from losing weight.

- **Do keep daily sodium intake under 1,200mg.**
  A low-salt diet can help to avoid water retention and bloating.

Eat when you want

- **Do honor your hunger signals and cravings.**
  It is important to let your body be your guide when eating (or not eating). Trust that it knows when you are hungry and when you are satisfied.

- **Do eat every 3 hours to keep your blood sugar levels stable.**
  Try not to go longer than four hours without eating. This will help you to avoid stuffing yourself later.

Know What You're Eating

- **Do cook for yourself.**
  This is the best way to ensure that meals are low fat, low sodium and contain only vegan ingredients.

- **Do check ingredient lists and food labels.**
  When buying packaged food, avoid anything with ingredients you can't pronounce or added fats, sugars, and sodium.

- **Do avoid common non-vegan ingredients.**
  Check the label for ingredients like gelatin, casein, lactose, lanolin, and whey.

Stay Curious and Creative

- **Do make note of the foods you eat and how your body reacts to them.**
  Everyone is different, and your body might not respond well to certain vegan ingredients. It's helpful to know what might be causing undesirable effects so you can quickly identify the problem rather than ditching a vegan diet altogether.

- **Do allow your body to adjust to legumes and high-fiber foods slowly.**
  When you're not used to eating beans, they can wreak havoc on your digestion if you eat too much too soon. Start with small portions and stay aware of how certain legumes make you feel.

- **Do get creative and experiment with healthy vegan recipes.**
  There are plenty of vegan blogs and websites dedicated to sharing raw and whole food recipes that are delicious and will help you feel amazing.

- **Do try vegan milk substitutes like rice, almond, and soy milk.**
  However, be aware that many of these milks contain added sugar, so buy the unsweetened version whenever possible.

- **Do substitute animal ingredients in recipes with vegan ones.**
  Common substitutes include applesauce, bananas, and ground flax seed for eggs and vegetable oil or milk substitutes for dairy.

Vegan Don'ts

Stay Away from Packages

- **Don't eat too many packaged meat substitutes which could prevent losing weight.**
  Vegan diets are increasing in popularity, which means that there are more vegan food substitutes on the market. Eating them occasionally is okay, but too much-processed food is never great for your body and there are more wholesome, natural vegan food options out there.

- **Don't assume that vegan always means healthy.**
  There are tons of cookies, candies, and chips that are vegan. Chocolate chip cookie dough ice cream made with soy milk isn't going to be any better for your waistline than the dairy version, so steer away with the exception of an occasional treat.

- **Don't eat processed sugar and sweets too frequently.**
  Refined sugar is addictive and poisonous. Plus, too much sugar can make you cranky and cause your

energy to plummet. It is okay to eat it every once in a while, but it's definitely not a daily staple.

- **Don't eat empty carbs like white bread and other processed grains.**
They have the opposite effect of complex carbs as they spike your blood sugar and cause it to crash later.

- **Don't believe food marketing tactics.**
Companies that label their foods as natural, vegan, or fat-free are often just trying to trick you into buying processed junk. Remember, potato chips are technically "all natural and vegan" but definitely not a weight loss food. Check labels and look at the nutritional value of these foods before purchasing them.

Avoid Overwhelming Your Body

- **Don't eat too much fiber too quickly.**
If your body isn't used to a high-fiber diet, it can cause gas, bloating, and even constipation. Ease into it by combining high-fiber foods with more starchy produce and slowly add more fiber over time.

- **Don't eat too many "high-fiber" cereals and bars.**
  There are many high-fiber products out there, but they often contain a lot of unnecessary ingredients and added sugar. You're better off eating fruits, vegetables, and whole grains.

- **Don't consume too many artificial ingredients or additives.**
  These can mess with your body and brain chemistry, so it's best to steer clear of the weird stuff made in a lab or factory.

Common Nutrition Mistakes

- **Don't restrict carbs.**
  Carbs are energy, so not enough carbs equals too much sleepiness.

- **Don't overdo it on healthy fats.**
  Limit nuts, nut butters, avocados, and oil to a total of 20% or less of your daily diet.

- **Don't forget about protein.**
  While most people eat too much protein, not enough will have adverse effects like muscle waste and a weakened immune system.

- **Don't severely restrict your food intake — the cause of intense cravings and a slow metabolism.**
  Not all food is created equal, and to get enough calories vegans usually have to eat greater volumes of food. Not eating enough will slow down your metabolism and put your body into starvation mode, making it harder to drop pounds.

- **Don't forget to supplement your diet with B12 for more energy and a metabolism booster.**
  Humans need B12 and, unfortunately, most people get it from consuming animal products. Buy nutritional yeast to add to your food or purchase a daily B12 supplement at a pharmacy or health food store.

Emotional Pitfalls

- **Don't put foods into bad and good categories.**
  Telling yourself you can't eat something because it's bad will psychologically make you want it more, setting you up for food binges and guilty feelings. Eating a cookie doesn't make you a criminal and eating a salad doesn't make you a saint. Instead of tying complex emotions to your eating habits, focus on your body's natural cravings. Make it a goal to

savor the taste of nourishing foods and acknowledge their health promoting, satiating qualities.

- **Don't be too hard on yourself.**
Remember, transitioning to a vegan lifestyle is an ongoing process, so don't expect immediate perfection. There will be plenty of ups and downs, so be patient and enjoy your improvements and accomplishments along the way. Simply taking steps for a more healthy and compassionate life is enough cause for celebration!

Success Stories: Rice and Raw

Sasha

In 6 months she lost 30 pounds without restricting or count calories. In fact, she said she felt like she was eating too much food! She didn't even work out, but the weight just fell off on a high carb, low fat vegan diet filled with fruits, veggies, rice, and other whole foods. Check out her story:

http://bit.ly/1T68xzG

5 TIPS FOR WEIGHT LOSS TO GET VEGAN LEAN

1. **Low Sodium = Slimmer**

   Too much sodium can cause water retention making you feel bloated and sometimes too much salt can leave you feeling more hungry. Aim for fewer than 1,000 mg a day.

2. **Low Fat for a Lean Body**

   Although our body needs healthy sources of fat for easier digestion as well as a healthy body, too much fat can get stored causing weight gain. Shoot for fewer than 20% fat in your daily diet. To find out how to start knowing what your 20% is, you can log your foods for a few days into a calorie counter that also calculates the percentage of carbohydrates, fats, and protein.

3. 70% Plant-Based Meals for Fat Burning

This is the easiest trick to make sure your getting more fat burning, energizing, and nutrient-dense foods throughout the day and keeping your calorie in-take low. Plant-based means vegetables and fruits.

4. Go Green to Cleanse

Leafy greens are one of the best ways to keep you energized throughout the day and alkalize your body, which means they are best for releasing toxins and naturally cleansing the body.

5. B Vitamins for Booming Energy

A great natural source of b vitamins is in Kombucha tea. This drink has so many other benefits and helps with digestion from the natural probiotics. A glass of this drink every morning will have you ready to start the day that your morning coffee will look unnecessary.

5 DAY MEAL PLAN GUIDE FOR FASTER RESULTS

This is just meant to be a guideline but definitely check out some other high carb, low fat vegans on YouTube, pinterest, and other online sources. Check out what other vegans eat in a day to get ideas and creative, new recipes to try.

Helpful Tips:

Bloating Cure
Is caused by having too much fiber if your body is not used to it. Ease into this diet if it's too much on your digestion or try taking some vegan digestive enzymes.

Eat Slowly
This will also help with less bloating and proper digestion

Drink Lots of Water in Between Meals

Helps with digestion as well and reducing bloating

70% (or more) Water-Based Foods for Each Meal

The majority of your daily diet should be vegetables and fruits for the best results and the maximum energy throughout the day

Stick with It!

You will most likely lose weight easily but make sure you stick with this lifestyle so that you don't gain the weight back. Definitely check out other vegan lifestyle forums and videos to keep you inspired. However, with all the energy you'll have from all the carbs and natural nutrients you'll have a hard time going back to old ways.

Eat Until You're 80% Full

Restricting your calories only leads to getting extremely hungry at the end of the day or leads to binge eating on junk foods. Make sure for each meal you are satisfied by loading up on healthy carbs.

Keep Heavier, Cooked Meals for Dinner

Since fruit and veggies digest quickly, eat them earlier in the day for easier digestion and less bloating.

Day 1

Breakfast

First start your day with 2 big glasses of water

Energy Bursting Banana Smoothie
Spinach, kale, 1 tsp. of chia seeds, and bananas with water blended

Snack

Cucumber Mango Crisps
10-20 brown rice crackers (no salt crackers), cucumber slices, and mango slices

Lunch

Tropical Salad
1 banana (as appetizer) + big salad of greens, carrots, tomatoes, cucumbers, mango slices, ¼ avocado, and any other veggies your like with oil-free dressing

Snack

Peachy, Crispy, Creamy
Peach slices and celery sticks with oil-free hummus

Dinner

Healthy Fries! + Nutrient Dense Veggies

2 potatoes (cut into strips, baked until crisp) with 2 tbsp. of ketchup or low fat/low sodium dressing, plus 2 or more cups of steamed veggies or salad

Day 2

Breakfast

First start your day with 2 big glasses of water

Creamy Delicious Vitalize Smoothie
6-8 dates, 1 tsp. of chia seeds, 2 cups of fresh spinach, and 1/3 of a cucumber with water blended

Snack

Goodness All Wrapped Up
Veggie and fruit wraps (wrap lettuce, shredded carrots, cucumbers, apple slices in a nori wrap or rice wrap)

Lunch

Power Packed Veggie Soup
Vegetable soup (carrots, celery, peas, corn, potatoes, roasted onions, and mushrooms in a low sodium vegetable broth) with 10 (no salt) brown rice crackers

Snack

Cucumber Mango Crisps

10-20 brown rice crackers (no salt crackers), with cucumber, mango, and avocado slices

Dinner

Italian Slimming Feast

1 cup of quinoa or gluten-free pasta with low sodium tomato sauce, topped with your favorite steamed veggies

Day 3

Breakfast

First start your day with 2 big glasses of water

B12 Enhancing Tea!
Kombucha tea: Get some booming energy with natural b vitamins

Melon Morning Jumpstart
4 cups or more of your favorite melon (cantaloupe, honeydew, or watermelon)

Snack

"The Fill Up" Protein Shake
Plant-based protein powder with almond, coconut, or soy milk

Lunch

Energizing Salad
Big salad with your favorite veggies, ¼ of an avocado, apple slices, and oil-free dressing

Snack

2 cups of grapes

Dinner

Pot of All Good Nutrients
1 cup of white or brown rice with 3 or more cups of steamed veggies, and 1/3 cup of your favorite beans or lentils

Day 4

Breakfast

First start your day with 2 big glasses of water

Comforting Cinnamon Pear Oatmeal
½ cup of heated oatmeal (with water or dairy-free milk), pear slices (baked for 10 min), 1 tsp. of almond slices, raisins, and sprinkled cinnamon on top

Snack

Creamy, Crunch Wrap
Lettuce, shredded carrots, cucumbers, tomatoes, and oil-free hummus in a nori wrap or rice wrap

Lunch

Zucchini Pasta
Spiraled zucchini, topped with roasted tomatoes, caramelized onions, any other veggies you like, and low-sodium tomato sauce (sprinkle with nutrition yeast for a cheesy flavor and B12 energy)

Snack

Apple Crisp with a Twist

Apple slices warmed topped with 1 tbsp. of crushed walnuts, cinnamon, and 1 tsp of maple syrup

Dinner

Healthy Pizza

Low-fat, low-sodium dough (or make your own) with low-sodium tomato sauce, and top with broccoli, tomato, onions, or your favorite veggies

Day 5

Breakfast

First start your day with 2 big glasses of water

B12 Enhancing Tea!
Kombucha tea: Get some booming energy with natural b vitamins

Perfectly Healthy Parfait
Small portion of low-fat granola, small scoop of soy or coconut yogurt, topped with lots of blueberries, strawberries, and 1 tsp of almond slices

Snack

"The Fill Up" Protein Shake
Plant-based protein powder with almond, coconut, or soy milk

Lunch

Tropical Salad
1 banana (as appetizer) + big salad of greens, veggies, 1/3 avocado, and mango slices with oil-free dressing

Snack

Creamy, Crunch Wrap
Lettuce, shredded carrots, cucumbers, tomatoes and oil-free hummus in a nori wrap or rice wrap

Dinner

Cleansing Stir-Fry
1 cup of white or brown rice with 3 or more cups of stir-fry veggies (use minimal olive oil or coconut oil when cooking)

BONUS: HOW TO STOP FOOD CRAVINGS IN LESS THAN 5 MINUTES!

If you have trouble with overeating your favorite junk foods like chocolate, cookies, cake, chips, cereal, etc. and would love to learn a unique strategy that eliminates emotional food cravings in just a few minutes check out Christine (the Craving Fighter Queen) Magnarelli's free video at **PowerOverCravings.com**

- Stop cravings for your most tempting foods in minutes
- See for yourself how the taste and smell of the food is less appealing after using this technique
- Use this strategy any time you feel cravings come on
- Help with your weight loss results in a totally new way

TO YOUR SUCCESS!

Thank you again for buying this book!

I hope this book is able to guide you through your transition into a healthy vegan lifestyle. Use the information that you have learned here as a tool to lose weight, get energized, and feel amazing.

The next step is to begin your vegan journey. A lifetime of good health and happiness is waiting for you!

Finally, if you enjoyed this book, then I'd like to ask you for a favor. Would you be kind enough to leave a review for this book on Amazon? It'd be greatly appreciated!

Thank you and good luck on your vegan journey.

Printed in Great Britain
by Amazon